Contents

Break the Sugar Habit

Governments spend a fortune on programs aimed at making us lose weight. They tell us to eat less fatty food and exercise more. Meanwhile we fork over ever-increasing amounts on gym memberships, packaged meals, books, magazines and the advice of experts. Despite decades of this we are now fatter than at any other time in history.

Increasingly the signs are that sugar, or more specifically, fructose (the sugar in fruit, and one half of table sugar), is the culprit behind the obesity crisis.

The Important Sugars

There are only three important simple sugars: glucose, fructose and galactose. All of the other sugars you are likely to encounter in daily life are simply combinations of these three.

Glucose is by far the most plentiful of the simple sugars. Pretty much every food (except meat) contains significant quantities of glucose. Even meat (protein) is eventually converted to glucose by our digestive system. It's a pretty important sugar to humans, as it is our primary fuel – no glucose means no us.

Galactose is present in our environment in only very small quantities and is found mainly in dairy products in the form of lactose (where it is joined to a glucose molecule).

Fructose is also relatively rare in nature. It is found primarily in ripe fruits, which is why it is sometimes call fruit sugar. It is usually found together with glucose and it is what makes food taste sweet. As well as fruit, it's naturally present in honey (40%), Maple Syrup (35%) and Agave Syrup (90%).

Sucrose is what we think of when someone says table sugar. It's one half glucose and one half fructose. Brown sugar, caster sugar, raw sugar and Low GI sugar are all just sucrose.

A very new and deadly addition to our diet

In 1870, the only way you could eat a significant amount of fructose was to be the king of England or to come into the small fortune required to buy sugar or honey. But now every person in Australia is eating just around 50 kilograms of sugar (25 kilograms of fructose) a year.

Soft-drink and fruit juice consumption alone has increased by 30 percent in just the last two decades and two thirds of the adult population is now overweight or obese. Today our collective weight problem continues to accelerate in direct proportion to our consumption of sugar.

A slew of recent research makes it clear that as a species we are ill-equipped to deal with the relatively large amounts of sugar (and therefore fructose) we now consume.

The research shows we have one primary appetite-control centre in our brain called the hypothalamus. It reacts to four major appetite hormones. Three of these hormones tell us when we have had enough to eat and one of them temporarily inhibits the effect of the other three and tells us that we need to eat.

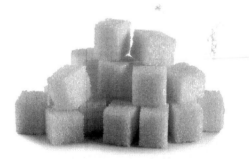

Fructose, uniquely among the food we eat, will not stimulate the release of any of the 'enough to eat' hormones. So we can eat it (and any food containing it) without feeling full. Worse still, fructose is not used for energy by our bodies. Instead all of the fructose is directly converted to fat by our livers. This means that by the time we finish our glass of apple juice (or cola or chocolate bar) the first mouthful will already be circulating in our bloodstream as fat.

Just to put the icing on the cake, recent research has now confirmed what most chocolate lovers have always suspected – sugar is as addictive as cocaine.

How to tell if you're addicted to sugar

Do you struggle to walk past a sugary treat without taking 'just one'?

Do you have routines around sugar consumption – for example, always having pudding or needing a piece of chocolate to relax in front of the TV or treating yourself to a sweet drink or chocolate after a session at the gym?

Are there are times when you feel as if you cannot go on without a sugar hit?

If you are forced to go without sugar for 24 hours, do you develop headaches and mood swings?

Obesity is just symptom of a litany of diseases caused by our fructose addiction. Some diseases are directly related to increased body weight, such as osteoarthritis, fractures , hernia and sleep apnoea. Some are related to the way in which fructose messes with our hormones, such as acne and polycystic ovary syndrome. Others are caused by the fructose induced flood of blood-borne fatty acids, notably cardiovascular diseases, fatty liver disease and type II diabetes. And recent research is also suggesting our overindulgence in fructose is directly linked to a variety of cancers, chronic kidney disease, erectile dysfunction and Alzheimer's disease.

Avoiding Fructose

The addictive ingredient in sugar is the fructose. And because it is addictive, food manufacturers have included it in just about everything.

Getting Fructose Out of Your Diet

Breaking a sugar addiction means that before you even start you've got to pick your way through a minefield of fructose filled foods. But in every category of foods there are some which are much lower in fructose than others. This Guide is all about helping you find those low fructose foods.

We know how difficult it is to stop smoking. Imagine how hard it would be if everything we ate or drank contained nicotine. Because much of our food is laced with fructose, breaking a sugar habit is far harder than giving up smoking. But if you use this guide to help with the shopping, you will have avoided most dietary fructose.

The rules for including a food are pretty simple:

1. **Drinks must have no fructose per 100ml.**

2. **Foods must have less than 1.5g of fructose per 100g (less than 3g per 100g of 'Sugars' on the label)**

The reason for the harsh limit on drinks is that we usually drink much more than 100ml at a time. A can of soft drink is 375 ml, a bottle is 600 ml and some fast food outlets serve soft drink in 1 litre sizes. Foods on the other hand are often served at or around the hundred gram mark (except yoghurts and ice-creams which are usually 200 g).

The label on the food is the primary source for information about fructose content. "Sugars" on the label are assumed to be sucrose (glucose + fructose) unless the ingredients list indicates otherwise. For example, dairy foods will often contain considerable quantities of lactose (galactose + glucose) which will appear under the heading 'Sugars'. Those foods have the probable lactose content deducted from the sugar's total before fructose content is calculated.

If a food is not in this list then it is either too high in fructose or I am not aware of it (please send me an email david@davidgillespie.org) to let me know about any missing foods.

Only processed foods are included in the list. If you plan to eat whole food only, then you don't need to know the sugar content, just keep fruit to a minimum (less than 2 pieces per day or 1 for a child). Juice or dried versions are not acceptable substitutes for whole fruit or vegetables.

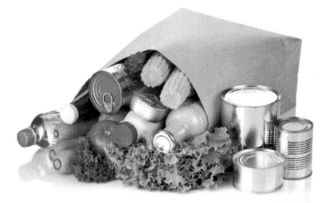

Sugar Substitutes

I'm not a big fan of the term artificial sweetener. It implies that other sweeteners (such as sugar, or fruit juice or high fructose corn syrup) are in some way natural, with all the goodness we have been conditioned to imply into that term. And there is nothing natural about extracting sugar from sugar cane. Substitute sweetener strikes me as a more appropriate description. They are substitutes for sugar, intended to do the job of sugar. In reality sugar itself is a substitute sweetener (for honey) but let's not get all technical. They are all created by using various levels of technology (from manmade beehives to industrial chemical plants) with the sole purpose of adding sweet taste to foods which are not otherwise sweet.

There are three categories of substitute sweetener; those that are absolutely safe to consume; and those that may be safe in limited doses and those which are not safe under any circumstances (usually because they are metabolized to fructose anyway).

Substitute Sweeteners commonly used in Britain

Good	Your call	Bad	
Corn Syrup	Acesulphame potassium (#950)	Agave Syrup	Mannitol (#421)
Dextrose	Alitame (#956)	Fructose	Maple Syrup
Glucose	Aspartame (#951)	Fruit Juice Extract	Molasses
Glucose Syrup	Aspartame-acesuphame (#962)	Golden Syrup	Polydextrose
Lactose	Cyclamates (#952)	High Fructose Corn Syrup	Resistant (malto) dextrin
Maltose	Erythritol (#968)	Honey	Sorbitol (#420)
Maltodextrin	Neotame (#961)	Inulin	Sucrose
Maltodextrose	Saccharin (#954)	Isomalt (#953)	Wheat dextrin
Rice Malt Syrup	Stevia (#960)	Lactitol (#966)	
	Sucralose (#955)	Litesse	
	Xylitol (#967)	Maltitol (#965)	

Seed Oils

The lists that follow are based entirely on sugar content alone. I have also written about the dangers of some types of vegetable oil (seed oils) in my book Toxic Oil. Some of the products in the lists below will contain seed oils, but as food manufacturers are not required to label the exact fats that they are using in a product, I have not included information about the fats in these lists. We can however have an educated guess and if you are concerned about the seed oil content of any product, I encourage you to use my fat ready reckoner chart available at www.howmuchsugar.com.

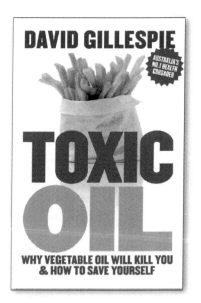

The Lists

Biscuits

Frozen Pizza

Ready Meals

Fast Food

Cereal Bars

No qualifying products.

The Atkins Advantage brand of bars are very low in sugar but use artificial sweeteners which are metabolized to fructose (the one's on the 'your call' list on previous page).

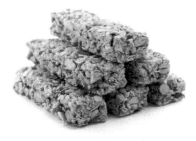

Drinks

The only qualifying products are unsweetened tea or coffee, diet soft drinks, water and milk (both whole and low fat).

The only branded soft drink which qualifies as low fructose is Lucozade Original. It is sweetened with glucose (only) and therefore contains no fructose.

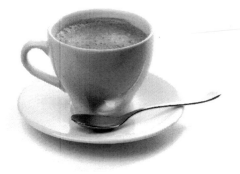

Confectionery

All of the following products have been sweetened with glucose rather than sugar (sucrose).

Maker	Product
Wonka (Nestle)	Runts
	Bottle Caps
	Everlasting Gobstopper
	Chewy Gobstopper
	Gobstopper Snowballs
Frusano	Filita Organic Whole Milk Chocolate
	Organic-Filita Amaranth
	Organic Rice-Crispies
	Filita Organic Dark Chocolate
	Organic Fili-Bears (Gummi Bears)
	Organic Blackberry Candies
	Organic Peppermint Candies
	Ricemalt peppermint hard candy
	Ricemalt lemon hard candy
	Ricemalt orange hard candy
	Dextrose Lolly

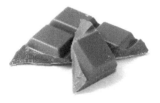

Condiments

These have been arranged by type and then by brand. You'll see that there are no options for some of the more common table sauces like Ketchup and BBQ Sauce. If you want those you'll have to make them yourself. I have provided some easy-to-make recipes in The Sweet Poison Quit Plan. All of these products contain seed oils except the Mustards and the ones marked with a * (yes, even the one that says it contains Olive Oil actually contains almost as much seed oil as the others).

Maker	Label	% Sugar
	MAYONNAISE	
ASDA	Real	2.6%
Heinz	Classic	2.9%
	Magnificent	2.9%
Hellmann's	Garlic	1.2%
	Real	1.3%
	with a touch of Garlic	2.2%
	Light	2.5%
	With a Zing of Lemon	2.5%
Morrisons	Plain	1.5%
	M Savers	2.2%
	Light	2.7%
Sainsbury's	Chilli	0.8%
	Plain	1.0%
	Thick & Creamy	1.0%
	French Style	2.0%
	Light	2.1%
	Organic	2.3%
Sainsbury's	Reduced Fat	2.7%
	Be Good To Yourself	2.9%

Maker	Label	% Sugar
Tesco	French	1.0%
	Plain	1.5%
	Real	1.5%
	Organic	1.8%
	Light	1.9%
	Finest Mayonnaise With Extra Virgin OliveOil	2.4%
	Finest Roast Garlic Cracked Black Pepper	2.7%
Winiary	Majonez	2.6%
MUSTARD*		
ASDA	Extra Special Tewkesbury	2.5%
French's	Classic Yellow	1.0%
Heinz	57	3.0%
Maille	Traditional Dijon	2.0%
	Wholegrain	2.0%
Morrisons	Dijon	1.1%
Sainsbury's	Wholegrain	1.6%
	Dijon	2.7%
	Horseradish	2.7%
Tesco	Dijon	1.0%
	Finest Wholegrain	2.2%
	Wholegrain	2.7%
SALAD CREAM & DRESSINGS		
ASDA	White Cooking Wine*	0.9%
Morrisons	Garlic Sauce	1.8%
Newmans	Italian Dressing	0.2%
Pizza Express	House Dressing*	2.7%
TABLE SAUCES		
Morrisons	Burger Sauce	3.0%

Cooking Sauces

These sauces are arranged by cooking style and then by maker and then by sugar content. Many of them contain seed oils (exceptions marked with a *). So be careful if you are also aiming to avoid them.

Maker	Label	% Sugar
	ASIAN	
ASDA	Chosen by You Red Thai Cooking Sauce	2.6%
	Chosen by You Thai Green Cooking Sauce	2.9%
Blue Dragon	Coconut Cream*	1.8%
Kingfisher	Coconut Milk Light*	1.0%
	Coconut Milk*	2.0%
Renuka	Coconut Milk*	0.0%
Sharwood's	Cantonese Curry Cooking Sauce*	2.9%
Thai Taste	Easy Thai Green Curry Kit*	1.1%
	Easy Thai RedCurry Kit*	1.1%
Tiger Tiger	Thai Green Curry Simmer Sauce*	1.9%
	INDIAN	
ASDA	Chosen by You Madras Cooking Sauce	1.0%
	Chosen by You Keralan Style Cooking Sauce	1.7%
	Chosen by You Fruity Biryani Oven Bake Sauce	2.1%
	Chosen by You Reduced Calorie Korma Cooking Sauce*	2.2%
	Chosen by You Balti Cooking Sauce	2.5%
	Chosen by You Indian Style Chana Dip	3.0%
Ashoka	Pav Bhaji*	0.7%
Loyd Grossman	Madras Sauce	2.7%

Maker	Label	% Sugar
Neesa	Chicken Balti Sauce	2.8%
Patak's	Madras Spice Paste	1.6%
Sainsbury's	Butter Chicken Curry Sauce	3.0%
Schwartz	Chicken Biryani Recipe Mix*	2.7%
Sharwood's	Lime Pickle Cooking Sauce	1.6%
	Vindaloo Cooking Sauce	2.6%
Tesco	Healthy Living Vegetable Rogan Josh Cooking Sauce	2.5%
	Saag Aloo Cooking Sauce	2.6%
	Tesco Spicy Lime Pickle	2.9%
ITALIAN		
ASDA	Chosen by You Reduced Fat Green Pesto	0.4%
	Four Cheese Pasta Sauce	0.8%
	Carbonara Pasta Sauce	1.1%
	Chosen by You Cheese & Bacon Pasta Bake	1.5%
	Smart Price Bolognese Sauce	1.7%
	Chosen by You Bechamel Sauce*	2.0%
	Chosen by You Green Pesto Sauce	2.2%
	Lasagne Topper	2.2%
	Chosen by You Parsley Simmer Sauce Mix*	2.5%
	Chosen by You White Simmer Sauce Mix*	2.5%
	Good for You Bolognese Pasta Sauce*	2.6%
	Chosen by You Spinach & Mascarpone Pasta Bake	2.8%
	Chosen by You Bolognese Sauce	3.0%
Dolmio	Express! Creamy Carbonara Pasta Sauce*	0.8%
	Express! Creamy Mushroom Pasta Sauce*	0.9%
	Carbonara Stir-In Sauce*	1.5%
	Pasta Bake Sauce for Macaroni Cheese	2.1%

Maker	Label	% Sugar
Dolmio	Cheesy Sauce for Lasagne	2.2%
	Carbonara Pasta Bake	2.5%
Homepride	Carbonara Pasta Bake	0.9%
	Ham & Mushroom Pasta Bake	1.9%
	Bolognese Sauce*	2.0%
	Cheese & Bacon Pasta Bake	2.1%
Loyd Grossman	Creamy Mushroom & Thyme Pasta Sauce*	0.2%
	Carbonara Sauce	0.9%
Morrisons	Green Pesto	0.4%
	White Lasagne Sauce	0.4%
	M savers Pasta Sauce	0.9%
Ragu	White Lasagne Sauce	1.9%
	Pasta Bakes Cheese & Bacon	2.2%
Sacla	Wild Rocket Pesto	2.3%
	Italian Tomato & Olive Pasta Sauce	2.7%
Sainsbury's	Pesto Alla Genovese, Taste the Difference *	0.1%
	Green Pesto, Light*	0.9%
	Pasta Sauce, Basics	1.8%
	Oven Baked, White Lasagne Sauce	2.0%
	Oven Baked, Macaroni Cheese	2.1%
Tesco	White Lasagne Pasta Sauce	0.1%
	Reduced Fat Green Pesto	0.4%
	Everyday Value Pasta Sauce (contains Saccharin)*	1.1%
	Creamy Peppercorn*	1.5%
	Spinach & Mascarpone Risotto Sauce*	2.2%
	Finest Pesto Alla Genovese*	2.2%
	Green Pesto	2.6%

Maker	Label	% Sugar
Tesco	Mexican	
Amoy	Reduced Fat Coconut Milk*	1.4%
Cofresh	Original Chilli Sauce*	1.5%
Dunn's River	Original Chicken Fry Mix*	0.4%
	Hot & Spicy Chicken Fry Mix*	1.0%
Old El Paso	Chunky Guacamole	1.1%
	Sliced Red Jalapenos*	1.3%
	Refried Beans	1.3%
	Sliced Green Jalapenos*	1.3%
	Cool Soured Cream Topping*	1.4%
	Enchilada Cooking Sauce	2.8%
Tesco	Refried Beans With Hint Of Lime*	1.0%
	Sour Cream Topping*	1.5%
	Everyday Value Chilli Con Carne Sauce*	2.5%
Weight Watchers	Chilli Con Carne Cooking Sauce*	2.7%
TRADITIONAL		
ASDA	Chosen by You Creamy Peppercorn Pour Over Sauce	0.2%
	Chosen by You Chasseur Cooking Sauce*	0.5%
	Chosen by You Red Wine Cooking Sauce	0.5%
	Chosen by You Instant Sauce Mixes Onion & Chive Sauce	0.9%
	Chosen by You Fish Pie Cooking Sauce	1.0%
	Chosen by You Instant Sauce Mixes Parsley Sauce	1.2%
	Chosen by You Instant Sauce Mixes Cheese Sauce*	1.3%
	Chosen by You Macaroni Cheese Pasta Bake	1.5%

Maker	Label	% Sugar
ASDA	Chosen by You Beef & Ale Slow Cook Sauce	1.6%
	Chosen by You Bourguignon Cooking Sauce	1.7%
	Chosen by You Beef & Ale Pour Over Sauce	1.8%
	Chosen by You Peppercorn Sauce Mix*	1.8%
	Chosen by You White Wine & Cream Cooking Sauce	1.8%
	Chosen by You Chicken Casserole Slow Cook Sauce*	2.3%
	Chosen by You Red Wine Pour Over Sauce*	2.3%
	Chosen by You Stroganoff Cooking Sauce	2.6%
	Chosen by You Gluten Free Cheese Simmer Sauce Mix*	3.0%
Chicken Tonight	French Country Chicken Chasseur & Red Wine Sauce	1.5%
	Creamy Mushroom Sauce	1.7%
	Rich & Creamy Mushroom Sauce	2.0%
	Classic Continental Country French White Wine Sauce	2.5%
Crosse & Blackwell	Country Chicken Casserole Sauce*	1.9%
	Cottage Pie Sauce*	2.5%
	Ale & Mushroom Casserole Sauce*	2.6%
Homepride	Beef Bourguignon Sauce*	0.9%
	Cheese & Ham Potato Bake	1.0%
	Garlic & Herb Potato Bake	1.1%
	Creamy Mushroom Chicken Sauce*	1.8%
	Creamy White Wine Sauce	1.9%
	White Wine & Cream Cook-In Sauce	2.4%
	Creamy Peppercorn Sauce	2.5%

Maker	Label	% Sugar
Homepride	Chicken Chasseur Sauce	2.6%
	Roast Chicken Casserole Sauce *	3.0%
Morrisons	White Wine Sauce	1.8%
Sainsbury's	Creamy Mushroom Cooking Sauce	1.6%
	Creamy Cheese & Bacon Potato Bake	1.7%
Sainsbury's	Oven Bake, Creamy Bacon & Leek	1.7%
	Beef & Ale Casserole Cooking Sauce	1.8%
	Dauphinoise Potato Bake	2.1%
	Cottage Pie Cooking Sauce	2.2%
Schwartz	Cheddar Cheese Sauce Mix	0.4%
	Creamy Watercress & Stilton Sauce*	0.4%
	Dauphinoise Potato Bake Recipe Mix	0.7%
	Classic Hollandaise Sauce for Fish*	0.7%
	Hollandaise Sauce Mix	0.8%
	Garlic, Mushroom & Cream Sauce Mix	1.2%
	Lasagne Mix*	1.2%
	Creamy Parsley Sauce Mix*	1.5%
	Chicken Casserole Sauce Mix	1.7%
	Creamy Pepper Sauce Mix	1.7%
	Spaghetti Carbonara Mi	2.0%
	Chicken & Leek Bake Mix	2.1%
	Creamy Mild Peppercorn Sauce	2.1%
	Savoury Mince Mix	2.4%
	Hot Chilli Con Carne Sauce Mix*	2.7%
Tesco	Dauphinoise	2.8%

Breakfast Cereals

I've presented this list in two formats so you can browse by sugar content or brand.

Breakfast Cereals – by sugar content

Label	% Sugar
Sainsbury's Puffed Wheat	0.5%
Sainsbury's Wholegrain Mini Wheats	0.6%
Nestlé Shredded Wheat Bitesize	0.7%
Shredded Wheat	0.7%
Kallo Gluten Free Original Puffed Rice	0.7%
Sainsbury's Scottish Oats With Whitebran & Oatbran	0.9%
ASDA Free From Pure Porridge Oats	1.0%
ASDA Ready Oats	1.0%
Jordans Organic Porridge Oats	1.0%
Quaker Oat So Simple Original Porridge	1.0%
Ready Brek Oat Cereal	1.0%
Sainsbury's Express Porridge Original	1.0%
Sainsbury's Instant Porridge, So Organic	1.0%
Sainsbury's Porridge Oats	1.0%
Sainsbury's Ready Oat Cereal	1.0%
Sainsbury's Scottish Porridge Oats	1.0%
Morrisons Instant Hot Oats	1.0%
Morrisons Porridge Oats	1.0%
M savers Oats	1.0%
ASDA Scottish Porridge Oats	1.1%

Breakfast Cereals - by sugar content (continued)

Label	% Sugar
Mornflake Medium Oatmeal	1.1%
Quaker Porridge Oats	1.1%
Sainsbury's Oat Flakes, Organic	1.1%
Sainsbury's Whole, Rolled Porridge Oats	1.1%
Scott's Old Fashioned Porridge Oats	1.1%
Scott's Porridge Oats	1.1%
Mornflake Oat Bran Sprinkles	1.2%
Mornflake Oatbran	1.2%
Flahavan's Organic Jumbo Oats	1.3%
Whitworths Seed Mix Topper	1.3%
ASDA Original Porridge Oats	1.5%
Good Grain Puffed Wheat	2.0%
Tesco Wholefoods Pure Oatbran	2.1%
Jordans Natural Bran	2.3%
Sainsbury's Wholewheat Biscuits, Basics	2.5%
M savers Wheat Biscuits	2.5%

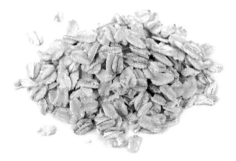

Breakfast Cereals - alphabetical

Brand	Label	% Sugar
ASDA	ASDA Free From Pure Porridge Oats	1.0%
	ASDA Original Porridge Oats	1.5%
	ASDA Ready Oats	1.0%
	ASDA Scottish Porridge Oats	1.1%
Flahavan's	Flahavan's Organic Jumbo Oats	1.3%
Good Grain	Good Grain Puffed Wheat	2.0%
Jordans	Jordans Natural Bran	2.3%
	Jordans Organic Porridge Oats	1.0%
Kallo	Kallo Gluten Free Original Puffed Rice	0.7%
M (Morrisons)	M savers Oats	1.0%
	M savers Wheat Biscuits	2.5%
Mornflake	Mornflake Medium Oatmeal	1.1%
	Mornflake Oat Bran Sprinkles	1.2%
	Mornflake Oatbran	1.2%
Morrisons	Morrisons Instant Hot Oats	1.0%
	Morrisons Porridge Oats	1.0%
Nestlé	Nestlé Shredded Wheat	0.7%
	Nestlé Shredded Wheat Bitesize	0.7%
Quaker	Quaker Oat So Simple Original Porridge	1.0%
	Quaker Porridge Oats	1.1%
Ready Brek	Ready Brek Oat Cereal	1.0%
Sainsbury's	Sainsbury's Express Porridge Original	1.0%
	Sainsbury's Instant Porridge, So Organic	1.0%
	Sainsbury's Oat Flakes, Organic	1.1%
	Sainsbury's Porridge Oats	1.0%
	Sainsbury's Puffed Wheat	0.5%

Breakfast Cereals - alphabetical (continued)

Brand	Label	% Sugar
	Sainsbury's Ready Oat Cereal	1.0%
	Sainsbury's Scottish Oats With Whitebran & Oatbran	0.9%
	Sainsbury's Scottish Porridge Oats	1.0%
	Sainsbury's Whole, Rolled Porridge Oats	1.1%
	Sainsbury's Wholegrain Mini Wheats	0.6%
	Sainsbury's Wholewheat Biscuits, Basics	2.5%
Scott's	Scott's Old Fashioned Porridge Oats	1.1%
	Scott's Porridge Oats	1.1%
Tesco	Tesco Wholefoods Pure Oatbran	2.1%
Whitworths	Whitworths Seed Mix Topper	1.3%

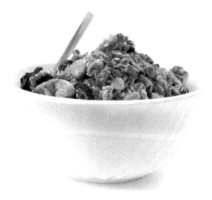

Ice-Cream

You won't be surprised to find that there no store bought ice-creams
which satisfy the rule. Even a small bowl (200 g) of the lowest-sugar ice-cream
(Weight Watchers Toffee & Honeycomb Sundae) delivers four teaspoons
of added sugar. You'll be pleased to discover that I do provide a great recipe
for sugar-free ice-cream in the recipe sections of howmuchsugar.com, in
the Quit Plan Cookbook and in the Sweet Poison Quit Plan. Unfortunately,
however, you have to make it yourself; no manufacturer yet makes
ice-cream this way.)

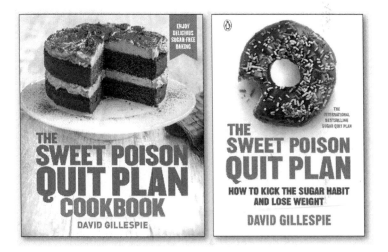

Yoghurts

I've presented this list in two formats so you can browse by sugar content or brand. You'll see that I've used a column called 'Adjusted Sugar'. This is a calculated amount based on removing the 4.7 grams of lactose that the typical yogurt contains. Lactose is a galactose molecule joined to a glucose molecule. The galactose molecule is metabolised to glucose by your liver and lactose is therefore essentially pure glucose and fructose free. Lactose does not count towards your 3g per 100g limit.

Yoghurts - by sugar content

Label	Adjusted Sugar
ASDA Extra Special Authentic Greek Yogurt	0.0%
ASDA Extra Special Fat Free Authentic Greek Yogurt	0.0%
Benecol Tropical Fruit & Soya	0.0%
Alpro Simply Plain Yogurt Alternative	0.0%
Benecol Dairy Free Mixed Berries	0.0%
Actimel 0.1% Raspberry	0.0%
Onken Natural Yogurt	0.0%
Yakult Light Milk Drink	0.0%
Onken Low Fat Natural Yogurt	0.0%
Total Greek Yogurts 170G	0.0%
Onken Low Fat Natural Yogurt	0.0%
Tesco Everyday Health 0% Strawberry Yogurt Drink 6x100g	0.0%
Total 0% Fat Greek Yogurt 500G	0.0%
Sainsbury's 0.1% Fat Normandy Natural Fromage Frais	0.0%
Onken Fat Free Natural Yogurt	0.0%

Yoghurts - by sugar content (continued)

Label	Adjusted Sugar
Benecol Strawberry Yogurt Drink	0.0%
Flora Pro .Activ Pomegranate And Raspberry 7x100g	0.0%
Flora Pro.Activ Strawberry Yoghurt Drink 7x100g	0.0%
Flora Pro-Activ Health Drink Strawberry	0.0%
Flora Pro-Activ Pomegranate & Raspberry	0.0%
Flora Pro.Activ Original Yogurt Drink 7x100g	0.0%
ASDA Natural Set Yogurt	0.1%
Activia Natural Pouring Yogurt	0.2%
Weight Watchers Berry Fruits Fromage Frais	0.2%
Rachel's Organic Dairy Natural Greek Yogurt	0.3%
ASDA Natural Fromage Frais	0.3%
Morrisons Greek Style Yogurt	0.4%
Activia Bio Natural Yogurt	0.4%
Tesco Chol Red Light Original Yoghurt Drink 6x100g	0.4%
Weight Watchers Confectionary Yogurts	0.4%
Weight Watchers Citrus Fruits Yogurt	0.5%
ASDA Greek Style Natural Yogurt Fat Free	0.6%
M savers Low Fat Natural Yogurt	0.9%
Benecol Blueberry	1.0%
Benecol Yogurt Drink Peach & Apricot	1.2%
Activia Natural Yogurt Low Fat	1.6%
Weight Watcher Dessert Recipe Yogurts	1.6%
Yeo Valley Organic Creamy Natural Yogurt	1.8%
ASDA Greek Style Natural Yogurt	1.9%
Activia 0% Fat Raspberry	2.2%

Yoghurts - by sugar content (continued)

Label	Adjusted Sugar
Benecol Light Yogurt Drink	2.2%
Sainsbury's Low Fat Natural Yogurt, Basics	2.3%
Tesco Low Fat Natural Yogurt 500G	2.3%
Muller Light Chocolate	2.4%
Muller Light Vanilla & Chocolate	2.4%
Ski Smooth Seasonal Yogurt	2.6%
Morrisons Low Fat Greek Style Yogurt	2.8%
Plum Baby Organic Fromage Frais	3.0%
ASDA Fat Free Natural Yogurt	3.0%

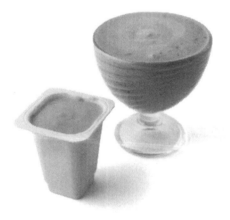

Yoghurts - alphabetical

Maker	Label	Adjusted Sugar
Actimel	Actimel 0.1% Raspberry	0.0%
	Activia 0% Fat Raspberry	2.2%
	Activia Bio Natural Yogurt	0.4%
Brooklea	Activia Natural Pouring Yogurt	0.2%
Chobani	Activia Natural Yogurt Low Fat	1.6%
	Alpro Simply Plain Yogurt Alternative	0.0%
ASDA	ASDA Extra Special Authentic Greek Yogurt	0.0%
	ASDA Extra Special Fat Free Authentic Greek Yogurt	0.0%
	ASDA Fat Free Natural Yogurt	3.0%
	ASDA Greek Style Natural Yogurt	1.9%
	ASDA Greek Style Natural Yogurt Fat Free	0.6%
	ASDA Natural Fromage Frais	0.3%
	ASDA Natural Set Yogurt	0.1%
Benecol	Benecol Blueberry	1.0%
	Benecol Dairy Free Mixed Berries	0.0%
	Benecol Light Yogurt Drink	2.2%
	Benecol Strawberry Yogurt Drink	0.0%
	Benecol Tropical Fruit & Soya	0.0%
	Benecol Yogurt Drink Peach & Apricot	1.2%
Flora	Flora Pro .Activ Pomegranate And Raspberry 7x100g	0.0%
	Flora Pro.Activ Original Yogurt Drink 7x100g	0.0%
	Flora Pro.Activ Strawberry Y oghurt Drink 7x100g	0.0%
	Flora Pro-Activ Health Drink Strawberry	0.0%

Yoghurts - alphabetical (continued)

Maker	Label	Adjusted Sugar
Flora	Flora Pro-Activ Pomegranate & Raspberry	0.0%
Morrisons	M savers Low Fat Natural Yogurt	0.9%
	Morrisons Greek Style Yogurt	0.4%
	Morrisons Low Fat Greek Style Yogurt	2.8%
Muller	Muller Light Chocolate	2.4%
	Muller Light Vanilla & Chocolate	2.4%
Onken	Onken Fat Free Natural Yogurt	0.0%
	Onken Low Fat Natural Yogurt	0.0%
	Onken Low Fat Natural Yogurt	0.0%
	Onken Natural Yogurt	0.0%
Plum	Plum Baby Organic Fromage Frais	3.0%
Rachel's	Rachel's Organic Dairy Natural Greek Yogurt	0.3%
Sainsbury's	Sainsbury's 0.1% Fat Normandy Natural Fromage Frais	0.0%
	Sainsbury's Low Fat Natural Yogurt, Basics	2.3%
Ski	Ski Smooth Seasonal Yogurt	2.6%
Tesco	Tesco Chol Red Light Original Yoghurt Drink 6x100g	0.4%
	Tesco Everyday Health 0% Strawberry Yogurt Drink 6x100g	0.0%
	Tesco Low Fat Natural Yogurt 500G	2.3%
Total	Total 0% Fat Greek Yogurt 500G	0.0%
	Total Greek Yogurts 170G	0.0%
Weight Watchers	Weight Watchers Dessert Recipe Yogurts	1.6%
	Weight Watchers Berry Fruits Fromage Frais	0.2%
	Weight Watchers Citrus Fruits Yogurt	0.5%

Yoghurts - alphabetical (continued)

Maker	Label	Adjusted Sugar
Weight Watchers	Weight Watchers Confectionary Yogurts	0.4%
Yakult	Yakult Light Milk Drink	0.0%
Yeo Valley	Yeo Valley Organic Creamy Natural Yogurt	1.8%

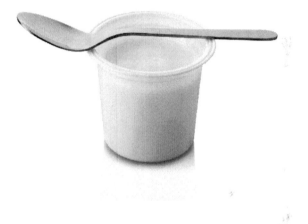

Breads

I've presented this list in two formats so you can browse by sugar content or brand. Almost all of the supermarket brands of bread contain rapeseed oil or another seed oil. If you are concerned about seed oil content then you will need to read the labels carefully. *Avoid any that say they contain 'Vegetable Oil'*

Breads - by sugar content

Maker	% Sugar
Sainsbury's Freefrom White Sliced	0.8%
Sainsbury's Sunflower & Pumpkin Seed SO Organic	1.4%
Warburtons Farmhouse White	1.6%
Genius Gluten Free Soft Brown	2.0%
Sainsbury's Multiseed Wholemeal	2.0%
Warburtons Toastie Sliced White	2.1%
Sainsbury's Freefrom Soft Brown Seeded	2.1%
ASDA Gluten Free Multi Seed	2.1%
ASDA Chosen by You White Medium Sliced	2.1%
Warburtons Medium Sliced White	2.1%
Tesco Stay Fresh Wholemeal	2.2%
Warburtons White Super Toastie Extra Thick	2.3%
Hovis Country Granary	2.3%
Hovis Nimble Wholemeal Sliced	2.3%
Warburtons Crusty	2.3%
Warburtons Crusty Premium White	2.3%
Warburtons Danish Sliced White	2.3%

Breads - by sugar content (continued)

Maker	% Sugar
Warburtons Medium Half And Half	2.4%
Sainsbury's Wholemeal Bread Medium Sliced, SO Organic	2.4%
Warburtons Half And Half Toastie	2.5%
Schneider Brot Organic Three Grain	2.5%
Hovis Soft White Medium	2.8%
Allinson Wholemeal Loaf	2.8%
Sainsbury's Wholemeal Bloomer	2.8%
ASDA Free From White Sliced	2.8%
Morrisons White	2.8%
Morrisons Wholemeal	2.8%
Vogel's Sunflower & Barley	2.9%
ASDA Extra Special Farmhouse Seeded Batch White	2.9%
Weight Watchers Danish White	2.9%
Hovis 7 Seeds Wholemeal	3.0%
Kingsmill Oatilicious	3.0%
Wheatfield Wholemeal	3.0%
Burgen Buckwheat & Poppy Seed	3.0%
Warburtons Seeded Batch	3.0%

Breads - alphabetical

Maker	Type	% Sugar
Allinson	Allinson Wholemeal Loaf	2.8%
ASDA	ASDA Chosen by You White Medium Sliced	2.1%
	ASDA Extra Special Farmhouse Seeded Batch White	2.9%
	ASDA Free From White Sliced	2.8%
	ASDA Gluten Free Multi Seed	2.1%
Burgen	Burgen Buckwheat & Poppy Seed	3.0%
Genius	Genius Gluten Free Soft Brown	2.0%
Hovis	Hovis 7 Seeds Wholemeal	3.0%
	Hovis Country Granary	2.3%
	Hovis Nimble Wholemeal Sliced	2.3%
	Hovis Soft White Medium	2.8%
Kingsmill	Kingsmill Oatilicious	3.0%
Morrisons	Morrisons White	2.8%
	Morrisons Wholemeal	2.8%
Sainsbury's	Sainsbury's Freefrom Soft Brown Seeded	2.1%
	Sainsbury's Freefrom White Sliced	0.8%
	Sainsbury's Multiseed Wholemeal	2.0%
	Sainsbury's Sunflower & Pumpkin Seed SO Organic	1.4%
	Sainsbury's Wholemeal Bloomer	2.8%
	Sainsbury's Wholemeal Bread Medium Sliced, SO Organic	2.4%
Schneider Brot	Schneider Brot Organic Three Grain	2.5%
Tesco	Tesco Stay Fresh Wholemeal	2.2%

Breads - alphabetical (continued)

Maker	Type	% Sugar
Vogel's	Vogel's Sunflower & Barley	2.9%
Warburtons	Warburtons Crusty	2.3%
	Warburtons Crusty Premium White	2.3%
	Warburtons Danish Sliced White	2.3%
	Warburtons Farmhouse White	1.6%
	Warburtons Half And Half Toastie	2.5%
	Warburtons Medium Half And Half	2.4%
	Warburtons Medium Sliced White	2.1%
	Warburtons Seeded Batch	3.0%
	Warburtons Toastie Sliced White	2.1%
	Warburtons White Super Toastie Extra Thick	2.3%
Weight Watchers	Weight Watchers Danish White	2.9%
Wheatfield	Wheatfield Wholemeal	3.0%

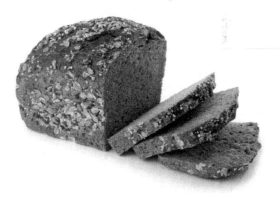

Biscuits

I've presented this list in two formats so you can browse by sugar content or brand. You might notice that all the biscuits in this list are essentially crackers. That's because the lowest sugar sweet biscuit you can get in Britain today is Sainsbury's Basics Shortbread Finger (12.8 percent sugar) and it's a long way outside the 3 percent rule.

Many of these biscuits will contain seed oils. If you are concerned about this, then use the fat reckoner chart available at www.howmuchsugar.com to determine whether your choice is likely to be as low in seed oil as it is in sugar.

Biscuits - by sugar content

Label	% Sugar
Morrisons Cheese Crispies	0.1%
Stockans Thin Oatcakes	0.3%
Morrisons Salt and Vinegar Rice Cakes	0.4%
Morrisons Rough Scottish Oatcakes	0.4%
Kallo Original Organic Wholemeal Rice Cakes	0.5%
Nairn's Cheese Oatcakes	0.6%
Tesco Rough Oatcakes	0.7%
Dr Karg Organic Emmental Crispbreads	0.8%
Marmite Rice Cakes	0.8%
Tesco Salt And Vinegar Cakes	0.8%
Tesco Lightly Salted Rice Cake	0.8%
Tesco Chive And Onion Twists	0.8%
Nairns Fine Milled Oatcakes	0.8%
Morrisons Cheesy Bites	0.9%

Biscuits - by sugar content (continued)

Label	% Sugar
Finn Crisp Original Crispbread	0.9%
Kallo Rice Cakes, Thick Organic Salted	0.9%
Nairn's Organic Oatcake	0.9%
Nairns Scottish Oatcakes	0.9%
Sainsbury's Cheddar Cheese Crispies	1.0%
Jacob's Cornish Wafer	1.1%
Nairns Gluten Free Oatcakes	1.1%
Nairns Gluten Free Cheese Oatcakes	1.1%
Morrisons Pizza Bites	1.2%
Carrs Melts Cheese Batons	1.2%
ASDA Good For You Rye Crispbreads	1.4%
ASDA Cream Crackers	1.4%
Jacob's Cream Cracker	1.4%
Jacob's Savours Salt & Black Pepper	1.4%
Sainsbury's Cream Crackers	1.4%
Carr's Water Biscuits	1.6%
Jacob's Cream Crackers High Fibre	1.6%
Sainsbury's Reduced Fat Cream Crackers	1.6%
Morrisons Dark Rye Crispbreads	1.7%
Snack A Jacks Salt & Vinegar	1.8%
Cypressa Cyprus Grissini Sticks	1.8%
Morrisons Salt & Pepper Bite	1.9%
Sainsbury's Parmesan & Basil Flatbread	1.9%
Sainsbury's 5 Seed Flatbread	1.9%
ASDA Chosen By You Tomato & Basil Melba Toasts	1.9%

Biscuits – by sugar content (continued)

Label	% Sugar
Nairns Seeded Oatcakes	2.0%
Llama's Baked Bites - Cheese	2.0%
ASDA Extra Special Italian Black Olive Breadsticks	2.0%
Sainsbury's Multiseeds Flatbread	2.0%
ASDA Gluten Free Crackerbreads	2.0%
ASDA Extra Special Italian Breadsticks	2.1%
Sainsbury's Poppy & Sesame Biscuit	2.1%
Doria Doriano Italian Crackers	2.2%
Sainsbury's Olive Oil Crostini	2.2%
Finn Crisp Original Rye	2.3%
Morrisons BBQ Flavour Rice Cakes	2.4%
ASDA Extra Special Olive Oil Ciappe	2.4%
ASDA Extra Special Rosemary Ciappe	2.4%
ASDA Cracker Snack	2.4%
ASDA Extra Special All Butter Green Olive Twists	2.4%
Weight Watchers Oat&Wheat Crackers	2.5%
Sainsbury's Oat & Thyme	2.5%
Krackawheat	2.6%
Morrisons Water Biscuits	2.6%
ASDA Gluten Free Lightly Salted Rice Cakes	2.7%
Snack A Jacks Prawn Cocktail	2.7%
Snack A Jacks Sweet Chilli	2.7%
DS Gluten Free Breadsticks	2.7%
M NuMe Tomato & Herb Wholegrain Snacks	2.8%
Fortts Original Bath Oliver	2.8%

Biscuits - by sugar content (continued)

Label	% Sugar
Sakata Tasty Japanese Rice Crackers, Sizzling Barbecue	2.8%
Kallo Sea Salt & Balsamic Vinegar Flavour Rice Cakes	3.0%
ASDA Cheese Twists	3.0%

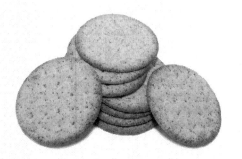

Biscuits - alphabetical

Maker	Label	% Sugar
ASDA	ASDA Cheese Twists	3.0%
	ASDA Chosen By You Tomato & Basil Melba Toasts	1.9%
	ASDA Cracker Snack	2.4%
	ASDA Cream Crackers	1.4%
	ASDA Extra Special All Butter Green Olive Twists	2.4%
	ASDA Extra Special Italian Black Olive Breadsticks	2.0%
	ASDA Extra Special Italian Breadsticks	2.1%
	ASDA Extra Special Olive Oil Ciappe	2.4%
	ASDA Extra Special Rosemary Ciappe	2.4%
	ASDA Gluten Free Crackerbreads	2.0%
	ASDA Gluten Free Lightly Salted Rice Cakes	2.7%
	ASDA Good For You Rye Crispbreads	1.4%
Carrs	Carrs Melts Cheese Batons	1.2%
	Carr's Water Biscuits	1.6%
Cypressa	Cypressa Cyprus Grissini Sticks	1.8%
Doria Doriano	Doria Doriano Italian Crackers	2.2%
Dr Karg	Dr Karg Organic Emmental Crispbreads	0.8%
DS	DS Gluten Free Breadsticks	2.7%
Finn	Finn Crisp Original Crispbread	0.9%
	Finn Crisp Original Rye	2.3%
Fortts	Fortts Original Bath Oliver	2.8%
Jacob's	Jacob's Cornish Wafer	1.1%
	Jacob's Cream Cracker	1.4%

Biscuits - alphabetical (continued)

Maker	Label	% Sugar
Jacob's	Jacob's Cream Crackers High Fibre	1.6%
	Jacob's Savours Salt & Black Pepper	1.4%
Kallo	Kallo Original Organic Wholemeal Rice Cakes	0.5%
	Kallo Rice Cakes, Thick Organic Salted	0.9%
	Kallo Sea Salt & Balsamic Vinegar Flavour Rice Cakes	3.0%
McVitie's	Krackawheat	2.6%
Llama's	Llama's Baked Bites - Cheese	2.0%
M (Morrisons)	M NuMe Tomato & Herb Wholegrain Snacks	2.8%
Marmite	Marmite Rice Cakes	0.8%
Morrisons	Morrisons BBQ Flavour Rice Cakes	2.4%
	Morrisons Cheese Crispies	0.1%
	Morrisons Cheesy Bites	0.9%
	Morrisons Dark Rye Crispbreads	1.7%
	Morrisons Pizza Bites	1.2%
	Morrisons Rough Scottish Oatcakes	0.4%
	Morrisons Salt & Pepper Bite	1.9%
	Morrisons Salt and Vinegar Rice Cakes	0.4%
	Morrisons Water Biscuits	2.6%
Nairn's	Nairn's Cheese Oatcakes	0.6%
	Nairns Fine Milled Oatcakes	0.8%
	Nairns Gluten Free Cheese Oatcakes	1.1%
	Nairns Gluten Free Oatcakes	1.1%
	Nairn's Organic Oatcake	0.9%
	Nairns Scottish Oatcakes	0.9%

Biscuits - alphabetical (continued)

Maker	Label	% Sugar
Nairn's	Nairns Seeded Oatcakes	2.0%
Sainsbury's	Sainsbury's 5 Seed Flatbread	1.9%
	Sainsbury's Cheddar Cheese Crispies	1.0%
	Sainsbury's Cream Crackers	1.4%
	Sainsbury's Multiseeds Flatbread	2.0%
	Sainsbury's Oat & Thyme	2.5%
	Sainsbury's Olive Oil Crostini	2.2%
	Sainsbury's Parmesan & Basil Flatbread	1.9%
	Sainsbury's Poppy & Sesame Biscuit	2.1%
	Sainsbury's Reduced Fat Cream Crackers	1.6%
Sakata	Sakata Tasty Japanese Rice Crackers, Sizzling Barbecue	2.8%
Snack A Jacks	Snack A Jacks Prawn Cocktail	2.7%
	Snack A Jacks Salt & Vinegar	1.8%
	Snack A Jacks Sweet Chilli	2.7%
Stockans	Stockans Thin Oatcakes	0.3%
Tesco	Tesco Chive And Onion Twists	0.8%
	Tesco Lightly Salted Rice Cake	0.8%
	Tesco Rough Oatcakes	0.7%
	Tesco Salt And Vinegar Cakes	0.8%
Weight Watchers	Weight Watchers Oat & Wheat Crackers	2.5%
	Woolworths Select Sea Salt Crackers	2.5%
	Woolworths Homebrand Water Cracker with Cracked Pepper	3.0%

Frozen Pizza

I've presented this list in two formats so you can browse by sugar content or brand.

Most of these frozen pizzas will contain seed oils. If you are concerned about this, then use the fat reckoner chart available at www.howmuchsugar.com to determine whether your choice is likely to be as low in seed oil as it is in sugar.

Frozen Pizza - by sugar content

Maker	Label	% Sugar
Morrisons	Garlic Pizza Bread	0.5%
Chicago Town	Deep Dish Chicken Melt	1.4%
Chicago Town	The Deep Dish Four Cheese Pizzas	1.5%
ASDA	Half & Half Combo Cheese/Pepperoni Pizza	1.5%
Chicago Town	The Deep Dish Meat Combo Pizzas	1.6%
Chicago Town	The Deep Dish Pepperoni Pizzas	1.6%
Tesco	Thin & Crispy Ham & Mushroom	1.8%
Chicago Town	Deep Dish Limited Edition	1.9%
Morrisons	Thin & Crispy Cheese & Tomato Pizza	2.0%
Trattoria Verdi	Thin Pepperoni	2.0%
Trattoria Verdi	Thin Cheese Pizza	2.1%
Morrisons	Thin & Crispy Pepperoni Pizza	2.1%
Sainsbury's	Pepperoni Pizza, Freefrom	2.2%
Tesco	Thin & Crispy Four Cheese	2.2%
Chicago Town	The Deep Dish Ham & Pineapple Pizzas	2.3%
Sainsbury's	Margherita Pizza, Freefrom	2.3%
Tesco	Thin & Crispy Pepperoni	2.3%
Dr Oetker	Ristorante Funghi	2.4%

Frozen Pizza - by sugar content (continued)

Maker	Label	% Sugar
Sainsbury's	Takeaway Meat Feast Pizza	2.4%
Morrisons	Takeaway Half 'N' Half Margherita & Pepperoni Pizza	2.4%
Morrisons	Takeaway Stuffed Crust Pepperoni Pile Up Pizza	2.5%
Panebello	Mozzarella Pomodoro	2.5%
ASDA	Half & Half Combo Ham/Spicy Chicken Pizza	2.5%
ASDA	Deep Pan Double Pepperoni Pizza	2.5%
Dr Oetker	Ristorante Speciale	2.6%
Sainsbury's	Stonebaked Pizza, Ham & Grilled Mushroom	2.6%
Sainsbury's	Thin & Crispy Margherita Pizza	2.6%
ASDA	Deep Pan Ham & Mushroom Pizza	2.6%
Morrisons	Deep Pan Cheese & Tomato Pizza	2.7%
Morrisons	Deep Pan Pepperoni Pizza	2.7%
Panebello	Carne Speciale	2.7%
Sainsbury's	Thin & Crispy Pepperoni Pizza	2.7%
Sainsbury's	Thin & Crispy Vegetable Pizza	2.7%
ASDA	Extra Thin & Crispy Mediterranean Vegetable Pizza	2.7%
Morrisons	Mighty Meatfeast Pizza	2.8%
Dr Oetker	Ristorante Pizza Mozzarella	2.8%
Trattoria Verdi	Topped To Edge Deep Cheese	2.9%
Chicago Town	Takeaway Four Cheese Pizza	3.0%
Chicago Town	Takeaway Pepperoni Pizza	3.0%
Goodfella's	Stonebaked Pizza, Extra Thin Crust, Pepperoni & Chorizo	3.0%
Sainsbury's	Stonebaked Pizza, Margherita & Pesto	3.0%

Frozen Pizza - by sugar content (continued)

Maker	Label	% Sugar
ASDA	Four Cheese Pizza	3.0%
Tesco	Deep Pan Four Cheese	3.0%
Trattoria Verdi	Topped To Edge Deep Pepperoni	3.0%

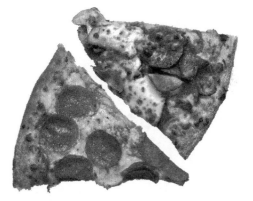

Frozen Pizza - alphabetical

Maker	Label	% Sugar
ASDA	Half & Half Combo Cheese/Pepperoni Pizza	1.5%
	Half & Half Combo Ham/Spicy Chicken Pizza	2.5%
	Deep Pan Double Pepperoni Pizza	2.5%
	Deep Pan Ham & Mushroom Pizza	2.6%
	Extra Thin & Crispy Mediterranean Vegetable Pizza	2.7%
	Four Cheese Pizza	3.0%
Chicago Town	Deep Dish Chicken Melt	1.4%
	The Deep Dish Four Cheese Pizzas	1.5%
	The Deep Dish Meat Combo Pizzas	1.6%
	The Deep Dish Pepperoni Pizzas	1.6%
	Deep Dish Limited Edition	1.9%
	The Deep Dish Ham & Pineapple Pizzas	2.3%
	Takeaway Four Cheese Pizza	3.0%
	Takeaway Pepperoni Pizza	3.0%
Dr Oetker	Ristorante Funghi	2.4%
	Ristorante Speciale	2.6%
	Ristorante Pizza Mozzarella	2.8%
Goodfella's	Stonebaked Pizza, Extra Thin Crust, Pepperoni & Chorizo	3.0%
Morrisons	Garlic Pizza Bread	0.5%
	Thin & Crispy Cheese & Tomato Pizza	2.0%
	Thin & Crispy Pepperoni Pizza	2.1%
	Takeaway Half 'N' Half Margherita & Pepperoni Pizza	2.4%
	Takeaway Stuffed Crust Pepperoni Pile Up Pizza	2.5%

Frozen Pizza - alphabetical (continued)

Maker	Label	% Sugar
Morrisons	Deep Pan Cheese & Tomato Pizza	2.7%
	Deep Pan Pepperoni Pizza	2.7%
	Mighty Meatfeast Pizza	2.8%
Panebello	Mozzarella Pomodoro	2.5%
	Carne Speciale	2.7%
Sainsbury's	Pepperoni Pizza, Freefrom	2.2%
	Margherita Pizza, Freefrom	2.3%
	Takeaway Meat Feast Pizza	2.4%
	Stonebaked Pizza, Ham & Grilled Mushroom	2.6%
	Thin & Crispy Margherita Pizza	2.6%
	Thin & Crispy Pepperoni Pizza	2.7%
	Thin & Crispy Vegetable Pizza	2.7%
	Stonebaked Pizza, Margherita & Pesto	3.0%
Tesco	Thin & Crispy Ham & Mushroom	1.8%
	Thin & Crispy Four Cheese	2.2%
	Thin & Crispy Pepperoni	2.3%
	Deep Pan Four Cheese	3.0%
Trattoria Verdi	Thin Pepperoni	2.0%
	Thin Cheese Pizza	2.1%
	Topped To Edge Deep Cheese	2.9%
	Topped To Edge Deep Pepperoni	3.0%

Ready Meals

I've presented this list in two formats so you can browse by sugar content or brand.

Most of these ready meals will contain seed oils. If you are concerned about this, then use the fat reckoner chart available at www.howmuchsugar.com to determine whether your choice is likely to be as low in seed oil as it is in sugar.

Ready Meals - by sugar content

Maker	Label	% Sugar
Sainsbury's	Classic Chicken Supreme	0.0%
ASDA	Free From Tomato & Basil Penne Pasta	0.1%
Weight Watchers	Chicken & Mushroom Tagliatelle	0.3%
Weight Watchers	Salmon & Broccoli Melt	0.3%
Tesco	Chinese Chicken Chow Mein	0.3%
Birds Eye	Salmon & Dill Pastry Bakes	0.4%
Morrisons	M Kitchen Chicken Fried Rice	0.5%
Morrisons	M savers Sliced Beef & Gravy	0.5%
Dietary Specials	Sausage Rolls	0.5%
Jus Rol	Party Sausage Rolls	0.5%
McDougall's	Upper Crust Deep Filled Chicken Pie	0.5%
Weight Watchers	Chicken Curry	0.5%
Sainsbury's	Cottage Pie, Basics	0.5%
Sainsbury's	Italian Spaghetti Carbonara	0.5%
Birds Eye	Roast Beef In Gravy	0.6%
Weight Watchers	Ocean Pie	0.6%

Maker	Label	% Sugar
Weight Watchers	Chicken Hotpot	0.7%
Aunt Bessie	Tidgy Toads	0.8%
McDougall's	Upper Crust Deep Filled Chicken & Asparagus Pie	0.8%
McDougall's	Upper Crust Deep Filled Steak Pie	0.8%
Sainsbury's	Chicken & Mushroom Pie	0.8%
Sainsbury's	Chicken, Ham Hock, Leek & Tarragon Pies	0.8%
Weight Watchers	Chicken & Lemon Risotto	0.8%
Bisto	Shepherd's Pie	0.8%
Sainsbury's	Sausage Rolls, Basics	0.9%
Georgia's	Free From Fish Cakes	0.9%
Sainsbury's	Steak Pie	0.9%
Young's	Chip Shop Large Cod Fillet & Chips	0.9%
Young's	Chip Shop Large Haddock Fillet & Chips	0.9%
Sainsbury's	Minced Beef Hotpot, Be Good To Yourself	0.9%
ASDA	Italian Spaghetti Carbonara	0.9%
Tesco	Everyday Value 2 Cheese Omelettes	0.9%
Morrisons	M Kitchen Cumberland Pie	0.9%
Sainsbury's	Chicken & Gravy Pie	1.0%
Bisto	Bangers & Mash	1.0%
Tesco	Chicken & Mushroom Pie With Mash	1.0%
Morrisons	M savers Chicken Supreme	1.1%
Birds Eye	Puff Pastry British Steak Pies	1.1%
Weight Watchers	Beef Hotpot	1.1%

Ready Meals - by sugar content (continued)

Maker	Label	% Sugar
Sainsbury's	Classic Cumberland Pie	1.1%
Sainsbury's	Classic Shepherd's Pie	1.1%
Sainsbury's	Pub Specials Chicken in Red Wine & Thyme Sauce	1.1%
Tesco	Chicken With Potato Wedges	1.1%
Tesco	Creamy Cheesy Chicken Hotpot	1.1%
Tesco	Everyday Value Chicken Curry	1.1%
Tesco	Everyday Value Fisherman's Pie	1.1%
Tesco	Everyday Value Macaroni Cheese	1.1%
Morrisons	M Kitchen Chicken & Bacon Carbonara	1.1%
Morrisons	M Kitchen Beef Stew & Dumplings	1.2%
Young's	Cheddar Crusted Fish Bake	1.2%
Weight Watchers	Beef Lasagne	1.2%
Tesco	Classic Chicken Casserole With Mash	1.2%
Tesco	Everyday Value Cottage Pie	1.2%
Tesco	Everyday Value Shepherds Pie	1.2%
Sainsbury's	Pub Specials Steak & Ale Pies	1.3%
Mr Brains	Faggots	1.3%
Cook's	Pie 'n' Mash With Liquor	1.3%
Sainsbury's	Pub Specials Chicken & Bacon Risotto	1.3%
Tesco	Classic Chicken Supreme With Rice	1.3%
Tesco	Classic Cumberland Pie	1.3%
Tesco	Classic Minced Beef Filled Yorkshire	1.3%
Morrisons	M Kitchen Fishermans Pie	1.3%
Morrisons	M savers 2 Cheese Omelettes	1.3%

Maker	Label	% Sugar
Aunt Bessie	Cheese & Onion Potato Bake	1.3%
Sainsbury's	Jumbo Sausage Rolls	1.4%
Linda McCartney	Vegetable Farmhouse Pie	1.4%
Sainsbury's	Beef Curry with Rice, Basics	1.4%
Sainsbury's	Roast Chicken Dinner	1.4%
Birds Eye	Beef Noodle Stir Fry	1.4%
Bisto	Roast Lamb Dinner	1.4%
Tesco	Classic Chicken Dinner	1.4%
Tesco	Everyday Value Chicken Hotpot	1.4%
Tesco	Everyday Value Toad In The Hole	1.4%
Tesco	Indian Chicken Korma With Rice	1.4%
Tesco	Light Choices Chilli & Wedges	1.4%
Sainsbury's	Cheese & Spring Onion Crispbakes	1.5%
Sainsbury's	Beef in Gravy, Basics	1.5%
Birds Eye	Shortcrust Creamy Chicken Pies	1.5%
Birds Eye	Shortcrust Meat & Potato Pies	1.5%
Birds Eye	Steak Pies	1.5%
Sainsbury's	Beef Lasagne, Be Good To Yourself	1.5%
Sainsbury's	Macaroni Cheese, Basics	1.5%
Sharwood's	Chicken Curry with Rice	1.5%
ASDA	Indian Chicken Tikka Masala with Pilau Rice	1.5%
Young's	Luxury Ocean Pie	1.5%
Sainsbury's	Classic Chicken Hotpot Dinner	1.5%
Birds Eye	Traditional Beef Dinner	1.5%

Ready Meals - by sugar content (continued)

Maker	Label	% Sugar
ASDA	Chicken Curry With Rice	1.5%
Bisto	Roast Beef Dinner	1.5%
Bisto	Roast Chicken Dinner	1.5%
Heinz	Big Chicken Casserole with Chunky Potatoes	1.5%
Sainsbury's	Pub Specials Gammon Hock In A Cider Sauce With Mustard Mash	1.5%
Tesco	Classic Turkey Dinner	1.5%
Tesco	Everyday Value Bangers & Mash	1.5%
Tesco	Everyday Value Corned Beef Hash	1.5%
Sainsbury's	Steak Puff Pastry Slices	1.6%
Weight Watchers	Mexican Chilli Wedges	1.6%
Sainsbury's	Classic Gammon & Parsley Sauce	1.6%
Birds Eye	Fish & Chips Dinner	1.6%
ASDA	Spaghetti Bolognese	1.6%
Tesco	Everyday Value Cheese Burger & Chips	1.6%
Tesco	Indian Beef Madras With Rice	1.6%
Morrisons	M Kitchen Pork Sausages & Mash with Onion Gravy	1.6%
Morrisons	M savers Beef Curry & Rice	1.7%
Morrisons	Cocktail Sausage Rolls	1.7%
Sainsbury's	Creamy Chicken Puff Pastry Slices	1.7%
Birds Eye	Chicken Pies	1.7%
Young's	Salmon Pie	1.7%
Weight Watchers	Beef & Red Wine Casserole	1.7%
ASDA	Reduced Calorie Chicken Curry	1.7%

Ready Meals - by sugar content (continued)

Maker	Label	% Sugar
Sainsbury's	Fisherman's Pie	1.7%
Tesco	Beef In Red Wine With Gratin Potatoes	1.7%
Tesco	Classic Shepherds Pie	1.7%
Morrisons	M savers Chicken Curry & Rice	1.8%
Sainsbury's	Steak & Kidney Pies	1.8%
Young's	Cheesy Fish Pie	1.8%
Weight Watchers	Steam & Serve, White Fish & Trulli Pasta	1.8%
Sainsbury's	Chicken Curry, Be Good To Yourself	1.8%
Tesco	Cumberland Sausage & Mash With Gravy	1.8%
Tesco	Everyday Value Cauliflower Cheese	1.8%
Tesco	Everyday Value Chilli Con Carne & Rice	1.8%
Tesco	Everyday Value Minced Beef Hotpot	1.8%
Tesco	Everyday Value Spaghetti Bolognese	1.8%
Morrisons	M Kitchen Prawn Tikka & Rice	1.9%
Sainsbury's	Chicken & Vegetable Pies, Basics	1.9%
Amy's	Bean & Cheese Burrito	1.9%
Sainsbury's	Chicken Curry with Rice, Basics	1.9%
Sainsbury's	Minced Beef Hotpot, Basics	1.9%
Bisto	Beef Lasagne	1.9%
Sharwood's	Chicken Korma with Rice	1.9%
Sainsbury's	Lemon Chicken Risotto, Be Good To Yourself	1.9%
Birds Eye	Traditional Chicken Dinner	1.9%
ASDA	Chilli Con Carne	1.9%

Ready Meals – by sugar content (continued)

Maker	Label	% Sugar
Heinz	Big Pasta Bolognese, with Chunky Pasta	1.9%
Tesco	Light Choices Chicken Tikka Masala	1.9%
Sainsbury's	Cheese & Onion Puff Pastry Slices	2.0%
Linda McCartney	Vegetarian Mushroom & Ale Pies	2.0%
Young's	Admirals Pie	2.0%
Weight Watchers	Spaghetti Bolognese	2.0%
Sainsbury's	Chicken Madras with Rice	2.0%
Young's	Fisherman's Pie	2.0%
Sainsbury's	Roast Beef Dinner	2.0%
Tesco	Chicken Casserole With Cheesy Leek Mash	2.0%
Tesco	Classic Lamb Hotpot	2.0%
Tesco	Goodness Chicken Tomato Pasta	2.0%
Tesco	Italian Beef Lasagne	2.0%
Tesco	Light Choices Chicken Hotpot	2.0%
Morrisons	M Kitchen Chicken Enchiladas	2.0%
Morrisons	M Kitchen Chicken Tikka Masala & Pilau Rice	2.1%
Sainsbury's	Steak & Mushroom Pies	2.1%
Hungry Joe's	Chicken Tikka Naan & Chips	2.1%
Young's	Smokey Macaroni Fish Bake	2.1%
Weight Watchers	Red Thai Chicken Curry	2.1%
ASDA	Family Favourites Beef Lasagne	2.1%
ASDA	Beef Curry & Rice	2.1%
Sainsbury's	Pub Specials Creamy Peppercorn Chicken With Sautéed Potatoes	2.1%

Ready Meals – by sugar content (continued)

Maker	Label	% Sugar
Hungry Joe's	Mighty Meatball Pasta Feast	2.1%
Tesco	Classic Beef Dinner	2.1%
Morrisons	M Kitchen All Day Breakfast	2.2%
Sainsbury's	Roast Lamb Dinner	2.2%
Sainsbury's	Classic Lamb Hotpot	2.2%
Sainsbury's	Pub Specials Beef Lasagne	2.2%
Sainsbury's	Pub Specials Slow Cooked Beef In Red Wine With Gratin Potatoes	2.2%
Birds Eye	Chicken Korma with Rice and Naan Bread	2.2%
Birds Eye	Chicken Curry with Rice and Naan Bread	2.2%
Tesco	Everyday Value Beef Lasagne	2.2%
Georgia's	Mexican Bake	2.3%
Holland's	Pudding, Steak & Kidney	2.3%
Sainsbury's	Toad in the Hole, Basics	2.3%
Sainsbury's	Chilli Con Carne with Rice	2.3%
Sainsbury's	Classic Beef Stew & Dumplings Dinner	2.3%
ASDA	Prawn Curry & Rice	2.3%
ASDA	Beef Lasagne	2.3%
Birds Eye	Chicken Jalfrezi with Rice & Naan	2.3%
Birds Eye	Chicken Tikka Masala with Rice and Naan Bread	2.3%
Hungry Joe's	Chicken Curry with Rice & Naan	2.3%
Tesco	Light Choices Beef Lasagne	2.3%
Amy's	Gluten Free Vegetable Lasagne	2.4%
Weight Watchers	Chicken Chop Suey	2.4%

Ready Meals – by sugar content (continued)

Maker	Label	% Sugar
Sainsbury's	Chicken Jalfrezi With Pilau Rice	2.4%
Tesco	Classic All Day Breakfast	2.4%
Morrisons	M savers Tuna Pasta Bake	2.5%
Dietary Specials	Gluten Free Quiche Lorraine	2.5%
Heinz	Big Chilli Con Carne	2.5%
Tesco	Indian Chicken Tikka Masala With Rice	2.5%
Sainsbury's	Classic Liver & Bacon Dinner	2.6%
Heinz	Big Beef Hot Pot	2.6%
ASDA	Butter Chicken with Rice	2.6%
Tesco	Goodness Chicken & Potato Bake	2.6%
Tesco	Indian King Prawn Masala With Rice	2.6%
Morrisons	M Kitchen Chicken Jalfrezi with Pilau Rice	2.7%
Morrisons	M NuMe Beef Lasagne	2.7%
Morrisons	M savers Chow Mein Noodles	2.7%
Aunt Bessie	Toad In The Hole	2.7%
ASDA	Reduced Calorie Chicken Noodles	2.7%
Young's	Salmon Fillet Dinner	2.7%
Weight Watchers	Sweet Mango Chicken	2.7%
Sainsbury's	Beef Lasagne	2.7%
Sainsbury's	Chicken In Black Bean Sauce With Rice	2.7%
ASDA	Red Thai Chicken Curry with Coriander Rice	2.7%
Tesco	Light Choices Chicken Pasta Bake	2.7%
Morrisons	M Kitchen Chicken Korma & Pilau Rice	2.8%

Ready Meals - by sugar content (continued)

Maker	Label	% Sugar
Morrisons	M Kitchen Chicken In Black Bean Sauce with Rice	2.8%
Amy's	Indian Mattar Paneer	2.8%
Weight Watchers	Tomato & Basil Chicken	2.8%
Sainsbury's	Butter Chicken with Rice	2.8%
Birds Eye	Chicken Stir Fry	2.8%
ASDA	Italian Spinach & Ricotta Cannelloni	2.8%
Heinz	Big Meat Feast Pasta Bake	2.8%
Sainsbury's	Vegetable Pies	2.9%
Georgia's	Free From Lasagne	2.9%
Sainsbury's	Pork & Leek Sausages & Creamy Mash in Onion Gravy	2.9%
Tesco	Italian King Prawn Linguine	2.9%
Weight Watchers	Chicken Tikka Masala	3.0%
Sainsbury's	Spaghetti Bolognese, Basics	3.0%
Sharwood's	Chicken Tikka Masala with Rice	3.0%
ASDA	Italian Spaghetti & Meatballs	3.0%

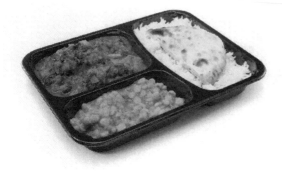

Ready Meals - alphabetical

Maker	Label	% Sugar
Amy's	Bean & Cheese Burrito	1.9%
	Gluten Free Vegetable Lasagne	2.4%
	Indian Mattar Paneer	2.8%
ASDA	Free From Tomato & Basil Penne Pasta	0.1%
	Italian Spaghetti Carbonara	0.9%
	Indian Chicken Tikka Masala with Pilau Rice	1.5%
	Chicken Curry With Rice	1.5%
	Spaghetti Bolognese	1.6%
	Reduced Calorie Chicken Curry	1.7%
	Chilli Con Carne	1.9%
	Family Favourites Beef Lasagne	2.1%
	Beef Curry & Rice	2.1%
	Prawn Curry & Rice	2.3%
	Beef Lasagne	2.3%
	Butter Chicken with Rice	2.6%
	Reduced Calorie Chicken Noodles	2.7%
	Red Thai Chicken Curry with Coriander Rice	2.7%
	Italian Spinach & Ricotta Cannelloni	2.8%
	Italian Spaghetti & Meatballs	3.0%
Aunt Bessie	Tidgy Toads	0.8%
	Cheese & Onion Potato Bake	1.3%
	Toad In The Hole	2.7%
Birds Eye	Salmon & Dill Pastry Bakes	0.4%
	Roast Beef In Gravy	0.6%

Ready Meals - alphabetical

Maker	Label	% Sugar
Birds Eye	Puff Pastry British Steak Pies	1.1%
	Beef Noodle Stir Fry	1.4%
	Shortcrust Creamy Chicken Pies	1.5%
	Shortcrust Meat & Potato Pies	1.5%
	Steak Pies	1.5%
	Traditional Beef Dinner	1.5%
	Fish & Chips Dinner	1.6%
	Chicken Pies	1.7%
	Traditional Chicken Dinner	1.9%
	Chicken Korma with Rice and Naan Bread	2.2%
	Chicken Curry with Rice and Naan Bread	2.2%
	Chicken Jalfrezi with Rice & Naan	2.3%
	Chicken Tikka Masala with Rice and Naan Bread	2.3%
	Chicken Stir Fry	2.8%
Bisto	Shepherd's Pie	0.8%
	Bangers & Mash	1.0%
	Roast Lamb Dinner	1.4%
	Roast Beef Dinner	1.5%
	Roast Chicken Dinner	1.5%
	Beef Lasagne	1.9%
Cook's	Pie 'n' Mash With Liquor	1.3%
Dietary Specials	Sausage Rolls	0.5%
	Gluten Free Quiche Lorraine	2.5%
Georgia's	Free From Fish Cakes	0.9%

Ready Meals - alphabetical

Maker	Label	% Sugar
Georgia's	Mexican Bake	2.3%
	Free From Lasagne	2.9%
Heinz	Big Chicken Casserole with Chunky Potatoes	1.5%
	Big Pasta Bolognese, with Chunky Pasta	1.9%
	Big Chilli Con Carne	2.5%
	Big Beef Hot Pot	2.6%
	Big Meat Feast Pasta Bake	2.8%
Holland's	Pudding, Steak & Kidney	2.3%
Hungry Joe's	Chicken Tikka Naan & Chips	2.1%
	Mighty Meatball Pasta Feast	2.1%
	Chicken Curry with Rice & Naan	2.3%
Jus Rol	Party Sausage Rolls	0.5%
Linda McCartney	Vegetable Farmhouse Pie	1.4%
	Vegetarian Mushroom & Ale Pies	2.0%
McDougall's	Upper Crust Deep Filled Chicken Pie	0.5%
	Upper Crust Deep Filled Chicken & Asparagus Pie	0.8%
	Upper Crust Deep Filled Steak Pie	0.8%
Morrisons	M Kitchen Chicken Fried Rice	0.5%
	M savers Sliced Beef & Gravy	0.5%
	M Kitchen Cumberland Pie	0.9%
	M savers Chicken Supreme	1.1%
	M Kitchen Chicken & Bacon Carbonara	1.1%
	M Kitchen Beef Stew & Dumplings	1.2%
	M Kitchen Fishermans Pie	1.3%

Ready Meals - alphabetical

Maker	Label	% Sugar
Morrisons	M savers 2 Cheese Omelettes	1.3%
	M Kitchen Pork Sausages & Mash with Onion Gravy	1.6%
	M savers Beef Curry & Rice	1.7%
	Cocktail Sausage Rolls	1.7%
	M savers Chicken Curry & Rice	1.8%
	M Kitchen Prawn Tikka & Rice	1.9%
	M Kitchen Chicken Enchiladas	2.0%
	M Kitchen Chicken Tikka Masala & Pilau Rice	2.1%
	M Kitchen All Day Breakfast	2.2%
	M savers Tuna Pasta Bake	2.5%
	M Kitchen Chicken Jalfrezi with Pilau Rice	2.7%
	M NuMe Beef Lasagne	2.7%
	M savers Chow Mein Noodles	2.7%
	M Kitchen Chicken Korma & Pilau Rice	2.8%
	M Kitchen Chicken In Black Bean Sauce with Rice	2.8%
Mr Brains	Faggots	1.3%
Sainsbury's	Classic Chicken Supreme	0.0%
	Cottage Pie, Basics	0.5%
	Italian Spaghetti Carbonara	0.5%
	Chicken & Mushroom Pie	0.8%
	Chicken, Ham Hock, Leek & Tarragon Pies	0.8%
	Sausage Rolls, Basics	0.9%
	Steak Pie	0.9%
	Minced Beef Hotpot, Be Good To Yourself	0.9%

Ready Meals - alphabetical

Maker	Label	% Sugar
Sainsbury's	Chicken & Gravy Pie	1.0%
	Classic Cumberland Pie	1.1%
	Classic Shepherd's Pie	1.1%
	Pub Specials Chicken in Red Wine & Thyme Sauce	1.1%
	Pub Specials Steak & Ale Pies	1.3%
	Pub Specials Chicken & Bacon Risotto	1.3%
	Jumbo Sausage Rolls	1.4%
	Beef Curry with Rice, Basics	1.4%
	Roast Chicken Dinner	1.4%
	Cheese & Spring Onion Crispbakes	1.5%
	Beef in Gravy, Basics	1.5%
	Beef Lasagne, Be Good To Yourself	1.5%
	Macaroni Cheese, Basics	1.5%
	Classic Chicken Hotpot Dinner	1.5%
	Pub Specials Gammon Hock In A Cider Sauce With Mustard Mash	1.5%
	Steak Puff Pastry Slices	1.6%
	Classic Gammon & Parsley Sauce	1.6%
	Creamy Chicken Puff Pastry Slices	1.7%
	Fisherman's Pie	1.7%
	Steak & Kidney Pies	1.8%
	Chicken Curry, Be Good To Yourself	1.8%
	Chicken & Vegetable Pies, Basics	1.9%
	Chicken Curry with Rice, Basics	1.9%
	Minced Beef Hotpot, Basics	1.9%

Ready Meals - alphabetical

Maker	Label	% Sugar
Sainsbury's	Lemon Chicken Risotto, Be Good To Yourself	1.9%
	Cheese & Onion Puff Pastry Slices	2.0%
	Chicken Madras with Rice	2.0%
	Roast Beef Dinner	2.0%
	Steak & Mushroom Pies	2.1%
	Pub Specials Creamy Peppercorn Chicken With Sautéed Potatoes	2.1%
	Roast Lamb Dinner	2.2%
	Classic Lamb Hotpot	2.2%
	Pub Specials Beef Lasagne	2.2%
	Pub Specials Slow Cooked Beef In Red Wine With Gratin Potatoes	2.2%
	Toad in the Hole, Basics	2.3%
	Chilli Con Carne with Rice	2.3%
	Classic Beef Stew & Dumplings Dinner	2.3%
	Chicken Jalfrezi With Pilau Rice	2.4%
	Classic Liver & Bacon Dinner	2.6%
	Beef Lasagne	2.7%
	Chicken In Black Bean Sauce With Rice	2.7%
	Butter Chicken with Rice	2.8%
	Vegetable Pies	2.9%
	Pork & Leek Sausages & Creamy Mash in Onion Gravy	2.9%
	Spaghetti Bolognese, Basics	3.0%
Sharwood's	Chicken Curry with Rice	1.5%
	Chicken Korma with Rice	1.9%

Ready Meals - alphabetical

Maker	Label	% Sugar
Sharwood's	Chicken Tikka Masala with Rice	3.0%
Tesco	Chinese Chicken Chow Mein	0.3%
	Everyday Value 2 Cheese Omelettes	0.9%
	Chicken & Mushroom Pie With Mash	1.0%
	Chicken With Potato Wedges	1.1%
	Creamy Cheesy Chicken Hotpot	1.1%
	Everyday Value Chicken Curry	1.1%
	Everyday Value Fisherman's Pie	1.1%
	Everyday Value Macaroni Cheese	1.1%
	Classic Chicken Casserole With Mash	1.2%
	Everyday Value Cottage Pie	1.2%
	Everyday Value Shepherds Pie	1.2%
	Classic Chicken Supreme With Rice	1.3%
	Classic Cumberland Pie	1.3%
	Classic Minced Beef Filled Yorkshire	1.3%
	Classic Chicken Dinner	1.4%
	Everyday Value Chicken Hotpot	1.4%
	Everyday Value Toad In The Hole	1.4%
	Indian Chicken Korma With Rice	1.4%
	Light Choices Chilli & Wedges	1.4%
	Classic Turkey Dinner	1.5%
	Everyday Value Bangers & Mash	1.5%
	Everyday Value Corned Beef Hash	1.5%
	Everyday Value Cheese Burger & Chips	1.6%
	Indian Beef Madras With Rice	1.6%

Ready Meals - alphabetical

Maker	Label	% Sugar
Tesco	Beef In Red Wine With Gratin Potatoes	1.7%
	Classic Shepherds Pie	1.7%
	Cumberland Sausage & Mash With Gravy	1.8%
	Everyday Value Cauliflower Cheese	1.8%
	Everyday Value Chilli Con Carne & Rice	1.8%
	Everyday Value Minced Beef Hotpot	1.8%
	Everyday Value Spaghetti Bolognese	1.8%
	Light Choices Chicken Tikka Masala	1.9%
	Chicken Casserole With Cheesy Leek Mash	2.0%
	Classic Lamb Hotpot	2.0%
	Goodness Chicken Tomato Pasta	2.0%
	Italian Beef Lasagne	2.0%
	Light Choices Chicken Hotpot	2.0%
	Classic Beef Dinner	2.1%
	Everyday Value Beef Lasagne	2.2%
	Light Choices Beef Lasagne	2.3%
	Classic All Day Breakfast	2.4%
	Indian Chicken Tikka Masala With Rice	2.5%
	Goodness Chicken & Potato Bake	2.6%
	Indian King Prawn Masala With Rice	2.6%
	Light Choices Chicken Pasta Bake	2.7%
	Italian King Prawn Linguine	2.9%
Weight Watchers	Chicken & Mushroom Tagliatelle	0.3%
	Salmon & Broccoli Melt	0.3%

Ready Meals - alphabetical

Maker	Label	% Sugar
Weight Watchers	Chicken Curry	0.5%
	Ocean Pie	0.6%
	Chicken Hotpot	0.7%
	Chicken & Lemon Risotto	0.8%
	Beef Hotpot	1.1%
	Beef Lasagne	1.2%
	Mexican Chilli Wedges	1.6%
	Beef & Red Wine Casserole	1.7%
	Steam & Serve, White Fish & Trulli Pasta	1.8%
	Spaghetti Bolognese	2.0%
	Red Thai Chicken Curry	2.1%
	Chicken Chop Suey	2.4%
	Sweet Mango Chicken	2.7%
	Tomato & Basil Chicken	2.8%
	Chicken Tikka Masala	3.0%
Young's	Chip Shop Large Cod Fillet & Chips	0.9%
	Chip Shop Large Haddock Fillet & Chips	0.9%
	Cheddar Crusted Fish Bake	1.2%
	Luxury Ocean Pie	1.5%
	Salmon Pie	1.7%
	Cheesy Fish Pie	1.8%
	Admirals Pie	2.0%
	Fisherman's Pie	2.0%
	Smokey Macaroni Fish Bake	2.1%
	Salmon Fillet Dinner	2.7%

Fast Food

Supermarkets aren't the only place you'll be buying food prepared by others. To cover off the majority of the market for 'restaurant' food, in this section, I've analysed the menu's of the major fast food chains.

WARNING: All fried food sold in these restaurants in Britain has been fried in seed oils and should be avoided if you are concerned about seed oils.

Subway Restaurants

Item	% Sugar
6-INCH BREAKFAST SANDWICHES	
Mega Melt	1.8%
Bacon	1.8%
Bacon, Egg & Cheese	1.8%
Sausage, Egg & Cheese	1.9%
Egg & Cheese	2.0%
Sausage	2.0%
BREAKFAST SUBS	
Mega Melt	2.3%
Sausage, Egg & Cheese	2.5%
Bacon, Egg & Cheese	2.7%
Sausage	2.8%

Subway Restaurants (continued)

Item	% Sugar
Bacon	2.8%
Egg & Cheese	3.0%
FLATBREAD SANDWICHES	
Chicken & Bacon Ranch Melt	1.4%
Chicken Temptation	1.6%
Tuna	1.6%
Spicy Italian	1.7%
Italian BMT	1.8%
Steak & Cheese	1.9%
Subway Melt	1.9%
Big Beef Melt	2.0%
Veggie Patty	2.7%
KIDS PAK SUBS	
Beef	2.5%
Turkey Breast	2.5%
Ham	2.8%
LOW FAT FLATBREAD SANDWICHES	
Chicken Teriyaki	1.7%
Chicken Breast	1.7%
Beef	1.8%
Turkey Breast & Ham	1.8%
Subway Club	1.8%
Turkey Breast	2.0%
Ham	2.0%
Veggie Delite	2.2%

Subway Restaurants (continued)

Item	% Sugar
Chicken Tikka	2.5%
Tandoori Chicken	2.7%
LOW FAT SUBS	
Subway Club	2.1%
Chicken Breast	2.2%
Beef	2.3%
Turkey Breast	2.3%
Turkey Breast & Ham	2.4%
Tandoori Chicken	2.5%
Ham	2.6%
Chicken Tikka	2.9%
REGULAR SUBS	
Chicken & Bacon Ranch Melt	1.8%
Chicken Temptation	2.0%
Tuna	2.1%
Spicy Italian	2.3%
Subway Melt	2.4%
Italian BMT	2.4%
Steak & Cheese	2.7%
Big Beef Melt	3.0%
SALADS	
Subway Club	1.3%
Chicken Breast	1.3%
Beef	1.4%
Turkey Breast	1.4%

Subway Restaurants (continued)

Item	% Sugar
Turkey Breast & Ham	1.4%
Chicken Tikka	1.5%
Ham	1.5%
Veggie Delite	1.5%
Chicken Teriyaki	2.1%
SIDES & SNACKS	
Garden Side Salad	1.6%
Melted Cheese Nachos	2.3%
SOUP	
Cream of Chicken	0.1%
Minestrone	0.2%
Highland Vegetable	0.3%
Country Chicken & Vegetable	0.4%
Wild Mushroom	0.5%
Lentil & Bacon	0.8%
Cream of Mushroom	0.9%
Beef Goulash	1.8%
Carrot & Coriander	2.4%
Leek & Potato	2.5%
Tomato	2.5%

McDonald's

Unfortunately there are no burgers under 3% sugar. The closest hamburger is the Nevada Grande (4.4%) or if you prefer chicken you can do slightly better with the Chicken Legend (3.5%). Here is a list of the items that are low in sugar.

Category	Item	% Sugar
Sides	Hash brown	0.0%
Chicken	Chicken Selects	1.1%
Sides	Fries	1.2%
Sides	Crisscuts	1.2%
Chicken	Chicken McNuggets	1.6%
Breakfast	Big Breakfast	2.0%
Breakfast	Double Bacon & Egg McMuffin	2.0%
Fish	Fish Fingers	2.1%
Breakfast	Double Sausage & Egg McMuffin	2.1%
Breakfast	Bacon & Egg McMuffin	2.3%
Breakfast	Sausage & Egg McMuffin	2.8%
Burger	Mighty Angus	2.9%
Burger	McChamp	3.0%

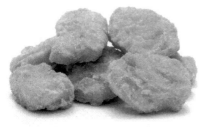

Burger King

The sugar content of most menu items at Burger King is surprisingly high in Britain. The only items that qualify are listed below. The lowest sugar beef burger you can buy is the Angus Smoked Bacon & Cheddar Double (4.2% sugar). Interestingly when you compare Burger King in the UK with its Australian equivalent (called Hungry Jack's for legal reasons), the differences in sugar content are remarkable. A Whopper in Australia is 2.3% sugar and would qualify for this list, but the same burger in Britain is 7.2% sugar.

Category	Item	% Sugar
Breakfast	Hash Browns	0.3%
Sides & Extras	Fries	0.4%
Sides & Extras	Satisfries	0.5%
Kids	Char-grilled Chicken Fillet Strips	1.6%
Sides & Extras	Chilli Cheese Bites (4 pieces)	1.8%
Chicken	Caesar Chicken Wrap	3.0%

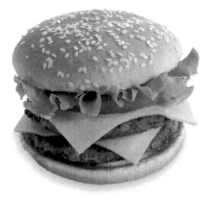

Pizza Hut

Note: These figures have not been adjusted for lactose (in the cheese) content as it is difficult to accurately estimate. All figures would be lower when adjusted for lactose.

Type	Size	Crust	% sugar
Premium Sides	BBQ Chicken Wings		0.1%
Classic Sides	Chips		0.1%
Premium Sides	Hot Dog Mini Bites		0.5%
Premium Sides	Chicken & Wedges Combo		0.6%
Premium Sides	Breaded Chicken Strips		0.7%
Premium Sides	Hot 'N' Spicy Chicken Strips		0.9%
Classic Sides	Potato Wedges		1.0%
Premium Sides	Cheese Triangles		1.1%
Premium Sides	Garlic Pizza Bread		2.0%
Pepperoni Feast	Medium	Pan	2.1%
Meat Feast	Medium	Pan	2.1%
Meat Machine	Large	Cheesy Bites	2.1%
Premium Sides	Macaroni Cheese		2.1%
Pepperoni Feast	Large	Stuffed Crust	2.2%
Pepperoni Feast	Large	Cheesy Bites	2.2%
Pepperoni Feast	Small	Italian	2.2%
Meat Feast	Large	Cheesy Bites	2.3%
Meat Feast	Large	Stuffed Crust	2.3%
Pepperoni Feast	Large	Pan	2.4%
Margherita	Medium	Pan	2.4%
Meat Feast	Large	Pan	2.4%

Pizza Hut (continued)

Type	Size	Crust	% sugar
Farmhouse	Medium	Pan	2.4%
Pepperoni Feast	Medium	Italian	2.4%
Super Supreme	Medium	Pan	2.4%
Meat Feast	Medium	Italian	2.5%
Margherita	Large	Stuffed Crust	2.5%
Margherita	Large	Cheesy Bites	2.5%
Farmhouse	Large	Stuffed Crust	2.5%
Hawaiian	Large	Stuffed Crust	2.5%
Meat Machine	Large	Stuffed Crust	2.5%
Farmhouse	Large	Cheesy Bites	2.5%
Hawaiian	Large	Cheesy Bites	2.5%
Super Supreme	Large	Stuffed Crust	2.5%
Super Supreme	Large	Cheesy Bites	2.6%
Meat Feast	Small	Italian	2.6%
Supreme	Medium	Pan	2.7%
Supreme	Large	Stuffed Crust	2.7%
Supreme	Large	Cheesy Bites	2.7%
Tuna Sweetcorn Melt	Large	Stuffed Crust	2.8%
Margherita	Large	Pan	2.8%
Chicken Supreme	Large	Stuffed Crust	2.8%
Farmhouse	Large	Pan	2.8%
Chicken Supreme	Large	Cheesy Bites	2.8%
Chicken Supreme	Medium	Pan	2.8%
Super Supreme	Large	Pan	2.9%
Margherita	Medium	Italian	2.9%

Pizza Hut (continued)

Type	Size	Crust	% sugar
Pepperoni Feast	Large	Italian	2.9%
Pepperoni Feast	Gluten Free		2.9%
Meat Feast	Gluten Free		3.0%
Premium Sides	Veggie Combo	3.0%	
Meat Feast	Large	Italian	3.0%
Farmhouse	Medium	Italian	3.0%
Margherita	Small	Italian	3.0%
Super Supreme	Medium	Italian	3.0%

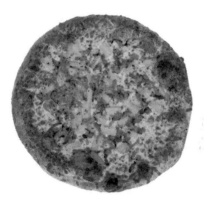

Domino's Pizza

There are no pizzas which qualify at Domino's in the UK. The sugar content ranges from 3.2% (Pepperoni Passion Double Decadence) to 16.9% (Italian Style BBQ Chicken Melt).

KFC

Category	Item	% Sugar
Meal	Original Recipe Snack Box	0.5%
Chicken	Hot Wing	0.5%
Chicken	1 Piece	0.5%
Meal	Bargain Bucket	0.5%
Meal	Hot Wings Snack Box	0.5%
Sides	Fries	0.5%
Meal	Popcorn Chicken Snack Box	0.5%
Meal	Mini Breast Fillet Snack Box	0.5%
Chicken	Mini Bucket	0.6%
Meal	Large Popcorn and 4 Regular Fries	0.7%
Sides	4 Piece Hot Shots	0.7%
Meal	Streetwise Mega Box	0.8%
Chicken	Mini Breast Fillet	0.8%
Chicken	Popcorn Chicken	0.9%
Sides	Secret Recipe Fries	1.1%
Meal	Boneless Banquet For One Box Meal	1.3%
Meal	Colonel's Bucket	1.7%
Meal	Wicked Variety Bucket	1.7%
Meal	Family Feast	2.6%
Sides	Gravy	3.0%
Meal	Fully Loaded Box Meal	3.0%
Meal	Streetwise Lunchbox	3.0%

Pret a Manger

Because there is quite a lot you can eat at Pret a Manger, I've provided the list in ascending order of sugar content and then a second version ordered by the category of food.

Category	Item	% Sugar
Sushi, Salad and Soup	Edamame Bowl	0.0%
Bakery	Artisan Soup Bread	0.0%
Sushi, Salad and Soup	Egg & Spinach Protein Pot	0.3%
Crisps	Rock Salt Popcorn	0.3%
Crisps	Maldon Sea Salt Crisps	0.5%
Sushi, Salad and Soup	Crayfish and Avocado No Bread	0.6%
Baguettes & Salad wraps	Smoked Salmon & Free Range Egg Breakfast Baguette	0.7%
Baguettes & Salad wraps	Free-Range Egg Mayo & Bacon Breakfast Baguette	0.7%
Baguettes & Salad wraps	Jambon-Beurre	0.8%
Sushi, Salad and Soup	Malaysian Chicken Curry Soup	0.8%
Baguettes & Salad wraps	Chicken Caesar & Bacon on Artisan	0.8%
Baguettes & Salad wraps	Wiltshire-Cured Ham & Greve Cheese Baguette	0.9%
Sushi, Salad and Soup	Crayfish & Quinoa Protein Pot	0.9%
Hot Food	Tuna Melt Toastie	1.0%
Sandwiches	Classic Ham & Eggs Bloomer	1.1%
Sushi, Salad and Soup	Tuna Nicoise Salad	1.1%
Sushi, Salad and Soup	Greens & Grains No Bread	1.1%
Bakery	White Soup Baguette	1.2%

Pret a Manger (continued)

Category	Item	% Sugar
Baguettes & Salad wraps	Italian Prosciutto on Artisan	1.2%
Sushi, Salad and Soup	Chicken, Broccoli & Brown Rice Soup	1.2%
Baguettes & Salad wraps	Posh Cheddar & Pickle on Artisan	1.2%
Hot Food	Ham, Cheese & Mustard Toastie	1.2%
Sushi, Salad and Soup	Mushroom Risotto Soup	1.2%
Crisps	Sea Salt & Organic Cider Vinegar Crisps	1.3%
Sushi, Salad and Soup	Grilled Asparagus & Prosciutto Salad	1.3%
Sushi, Salad and Soup	Aromatic Asian Chicken Soup	1.3%
Sandwiches	Free-Range Egg Mayo	1.4%
Sandwiches	Wild Crayfish & Rocket	1.4%
Sandwiches	Scottish Smoked Salmon	1.4%
Baguettes & Salad wraps	Brie, Tomato & Basil Baguette	1.4%
Baguettes & Salad wraps	Free-Range Egg Mayo & Roasted Tomato Breakfast Roll	1.5%
Sushi, Salad and Soup	Chef's Italian Chicken Salad	1.5%
Baguettes & Salad wraps	Pole & Line Caught Tuna Mayo & Cucumber Baguette	1.5%
Sandwiches	Chicken Avocado	1.5%
Sushi, Salad and Soup	Garden Pea & Mint Soup	1.6%
Sushi, Salad and Soup	Kale, Leek & Nutmeg Soup	1.7%
Sushi, Salad and Soup	Chicken, Edamame & Ginger Soup	1.7%

Pret a Manger (continued)

Category	Item	% Sugar
Sushi, Salad and Soup	Cream of Chicken Soup	1.7%
Sushi, Salad and Soup	Leek & Potato Soup	1.7%
Sushi, Salad and Soup	Pea & Ham Soup	1.7%
Sushi, Salad and Soup	Superfood Salad	1.8%
Sushi, Salad and Soup	Chef's Chipotle Chicken Salad	1.8%
Sandwiches	Eggs Florentine Bloomer	1.8%
Sandwiches	Kid's Cheese Sandwich	1.8%
Sandwiches	Kid's Ham Sandwich	1.8%
Hot Food	British Bacon Breakfast Roll	1.8%
Sandwiches	Classic Super Club	1.8%
Baguettes & Salad wraps	Grilled Asparagus, Herb & Nut Pesto on Artisan	1.9%
Hot Food	British Sausage & Egg Roll	1.9%
Sushi, Salad and Soup	Thai Chicken Curry Soup	1.9%
Sandwiches	Pole & Line Caught Tuna & Rocket Bloomer	1.9%
Sandwiches	Cracking Egg Salad	1.9%
Sandwiches	Wiltshire-Cured Ham & Pret Pickle	2.0%
Baguettes & Salad wraps	Avocado & Herb Salad Wrap	2.0%
Sandwiches	Mature Cheddar & Pret Pickle	2.0%
Hot Food	British Bacon & Egg Roll	2.0%
Baguettes & Salad wraps	Chunky Humous Salad Wrap	2.0%
Sandwiches	Super Greens	2.1%
Baguettes & Salad wraps	Chicken Sesame Sushi Wrap	2.1%

Pret a Manger (continued)

Category	Item	% Sugar
Hot Food	Italian Mozzarella & Pesto Toastie	2.1%
Sandwiches	Edam Salad	2.2%
Desserts & Pots	Porridge without Topping	2.2%
Crisps	Matured Cheddar & Red Onion Crisps	2.3%
Sushi, Salad and Soup	Peruvian Chicken Soup	2.3%
Sandwiches	Beech Smoked BLT	2.3%
Hot Food	Halloumi & Red Pepper Toastie	2.4%
Sushi, Salad and Soup	Pulled Pork Soup	2.4%
Sushi, Salad and Soup	South Indian Tomato & Spice Soup	2.4%
Baguettes & Salad wraps	Chicken Raita Salad Wrap	2.5%
Sandwiches	The New York Bloomer	2.6%
Sushi, Salad and Soup	Lentil & Bacon Soup	2.7%
Baguettes & Salad wraps	Lebanese Chicken Flat Bread	2.8%
Sushi, Salad and Soup	Carrot, Butternut & Spice Soup	2.8%
Sushi, Salad and Soup	Sausage Hotpot Soup	2.8%
Sushi, Salad and Soup	Flat Bread Mezze	2.9%
Sandwiches	All Day Breakfast	2.9%
Bakery	Ham, Bacon & Cheese Croissant	3.0%

Pret a Manger - by category

Category	Item	% Sugar
Baguettes & Salad wraps	Smoked Salmon & Free Range Egg Breakfast Baguette	0.7%
	Free-Range Egg Mayo & Bacon Breakfast Baguette	0.7%
	Jambon-Beurre	0.8%
	Chicken Caesar & Bacon on Artisan	0.8%
	Wiltshire-Cured Ham & Greve Cheese Baguette	0.9%
	Italian Prosciutto on Artisan	1.2%
	Posh Cheddar & Pickle on Artisan	1.2%
	Brie, Tomato & Basil Baguette	1.4%
	Free-Range Egg Mayo & Roasted Tomato Breakfast Roll	1.5%
	Pole & Line Caught Tuna Mayo & Cucumber Baguette	1.5%
	Grilled Asparagus, Herb & Nut Pesto on Artisan	1.9%
	Avocado & Herb Salad Wrap	2.0%
	Chunky Humous Salad Wrap	2.0%
	Chicken Sesame Sushi Wrap	2.1%
	Chicken Raita Salad Wrap	2.5%
	Lebanese Chicken Flat Bread	2.8%
Bakery	Artisan Soup Bread	0.0%
	White Soup Baguette	1.2%
	Ham, Bacon & Cheese Croissant	3.0%
Crisps	Rock Salt Popcorn	0.3%

Pret a Manger - by category (continued)

Category	Item	% Sugar
Crisps	Maldon Sea Salt Crisps	0.5%
	Sea Salt & Organic Cider Vinegar Crisps	1.3%
	Matured Cheddar & Red Onion Crisps	2.3%
Desserts & Pots	Porridge without Topping	2.2%
Hot Food	Tuna Melt Toastie	1.0%
	Ham, Cheese & Mustard Toastie	1.2%
	British Bacon Breakfast Roll	1.8%
	British Sausage & Egg Roll	1.9%
	British Bacon & Egg Roll	2.0%
	Italian Mozzarella & Pesto Toastie	2.1%
	Halloumi & Red Pepper Toastie	2.4%
Sandwiches	Classic Ham & Eggs Bloomer	1.1%
	Free-Range Egg Mayo	1.4%
	Wild Crayfish & Rocket	1.4%
	Scottish Smoked Salmon	1.4%
	Chicken Avocado	1.5%
	Eggs Florentine Bloomer	1.8%
	Kid's Cheese Sandwich	1.8%
	Kid's Ham Sandwich	1.8%
	Classic Super Club	1.8%
	Pole & Line Caught Tuna & Rocket Bloomer	1.9%
	Cracking Egg Salad	1.9%
	Wiltshire-Cured Ham & Pret Pickle	2.0%
	Mature Cheddar & Pret Pickle	2.0%

Pret a Manger - by category (continued)

Category	Item	% Sugar
	Super Greens	2.1%
	Edam Salad	2.2%
	Beech Smoked BLT	2.3%
	The New York Bloomer	2.6%
	All Day Breakfast	2.9%
Sushi, Salad and Soup	Edamame Bowl	0.0%
	Egg & Spinach Protein Pot	0.3%
	Crayfish and Avocado No Bread	0.6%
	Malaysian Chicken Curry Soup	0.8%
	Crayfish & Quinoa Protein Pot	0.9%
	Tuna Nicoise Salad	1.1%
	Greens & Grains No Bread	1.1%
	Chicken, Broccoli & Brown Rice Soup	1.2%
	Mushroom Risotto Soup	1.2%
	Grilled Asparagus & Prosciutto Salad	1.3%
	Aromatic Asian Chicken Soup	1.3%
	Chef's Italian Chicken Salad	1.5%
	Garden Pea & Mint Soup	1.6%
	Kale, Leek & Nutmeg Soup	1.7%
	Chicken, Edamame & Ginger Soup	1.7%
	Cream of Chicken Soup	1.7%
	Leek & Potato Soup	1.7%
	Pea & Ham Soup	1.7%
	Superfood Salad	1.8%

Pret a Manger - by category (continued)

Category	Item	% Sugar
	Chef's Chipotle Chicken Salad	1.8%
	Thai Chicken Curry Soup	1.9%
	Peruvian Chicken Soup	2.3%
	Pulled Pork Soup	2.4%
	South Indian Tomato & Spice Soup	2.4%
	Lentil & Bacon Soup	2.7%
	Carrot, Butternut & Spice Soup	2.8%
	Sausage Hotpot Soup	2.8%
	Flat Bread Mezze	2.9%

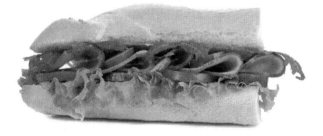

More Information

Still haven't found what you're looking for? I also maintain a database of over 2,000 foods including restaurant meals typically found in Asian and Mediterranean restaurants.

You can search the database for free at www.davidgillespie.org

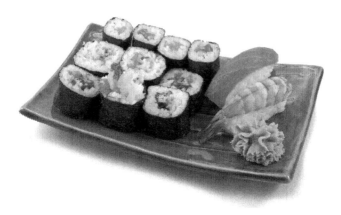

11584417R00049

Printed in Great Britain
by Amazon.co.uk, Ltd.,
Marston Gate.